Speech Therapy Works!
Juliana's Story

By Cynthia D. Sloan, MBA

ISBN: 978-1-950719-56-3 (Paperback)
ISBN: 978-1-950719-55-6 (eBook)

FIRST printing edition 2020.

J Merrill Publishing, Inc.
434 Hillpine Drive
Columbus, OH 43207

www.JMerrillPublishingInc.com

A message from Juliana

This book is written in honor of speech therapists in Ohio and all over the world. Especially the ones who helped me (Mrs. Seitz, Mrs. Bruner, and Mrs. Goldberg).

Thank you for helping kids like me! This is also written for kids who are receiving speech therapy or have graduated from the program. It is hard to go through a speech therapy program, but it is worth it.

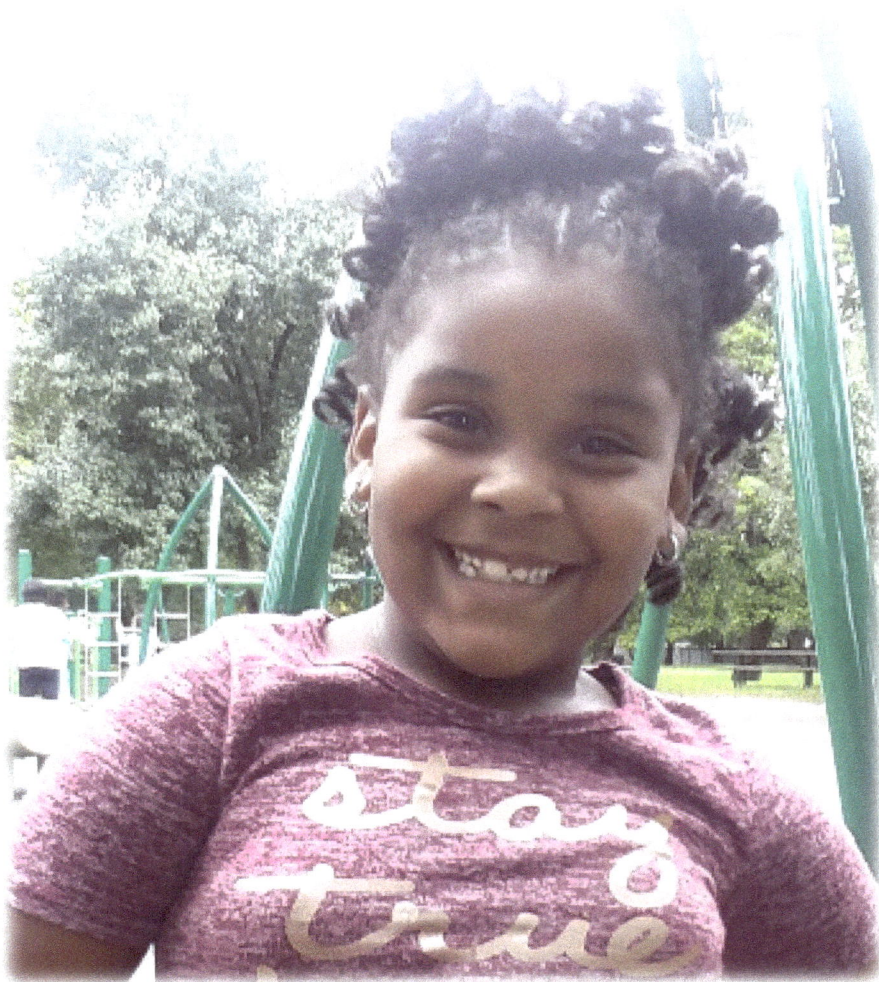

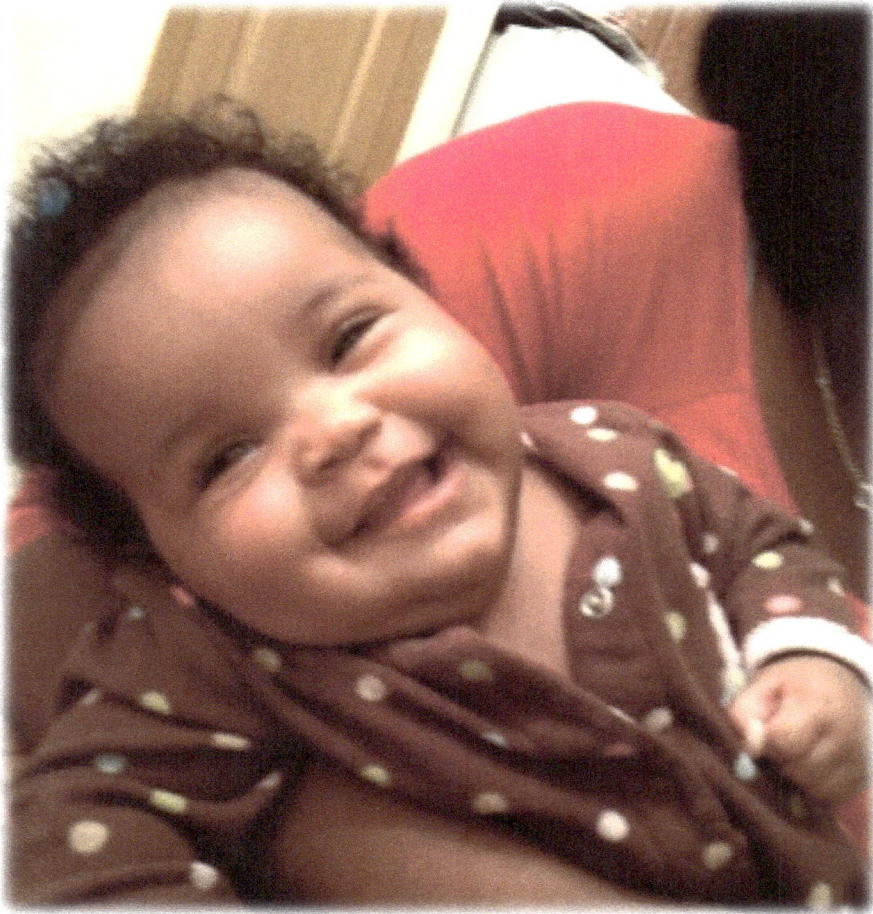

Juliana was a beautiful baby that constantly had a smile on her face! She was easy-going, calm, and friendly.

Juliana is my second daughter. We call her Julie or Jewels.

She enjoyed spending time with her big siblings: Jonathan, Jordan, Nathaniel, and Jenise.

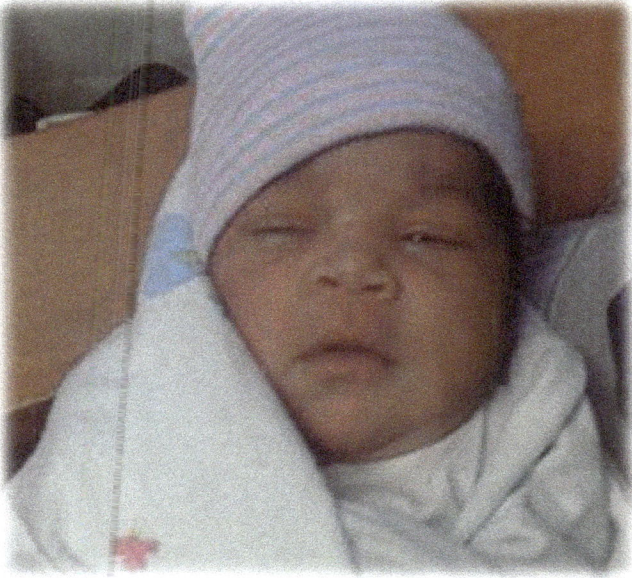
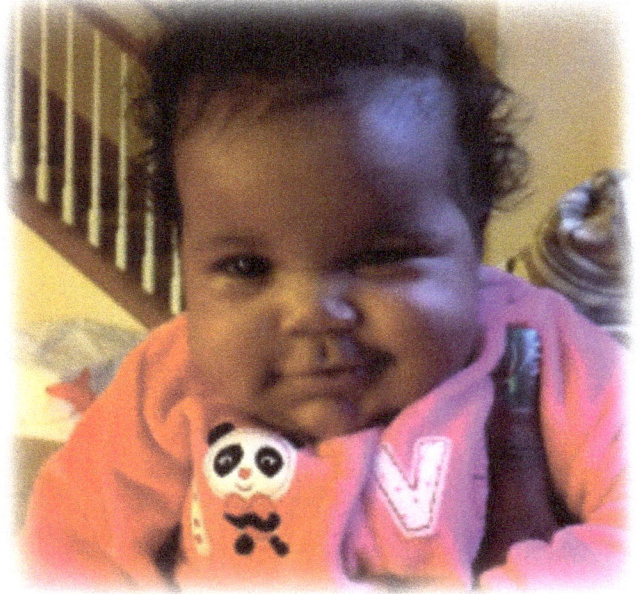
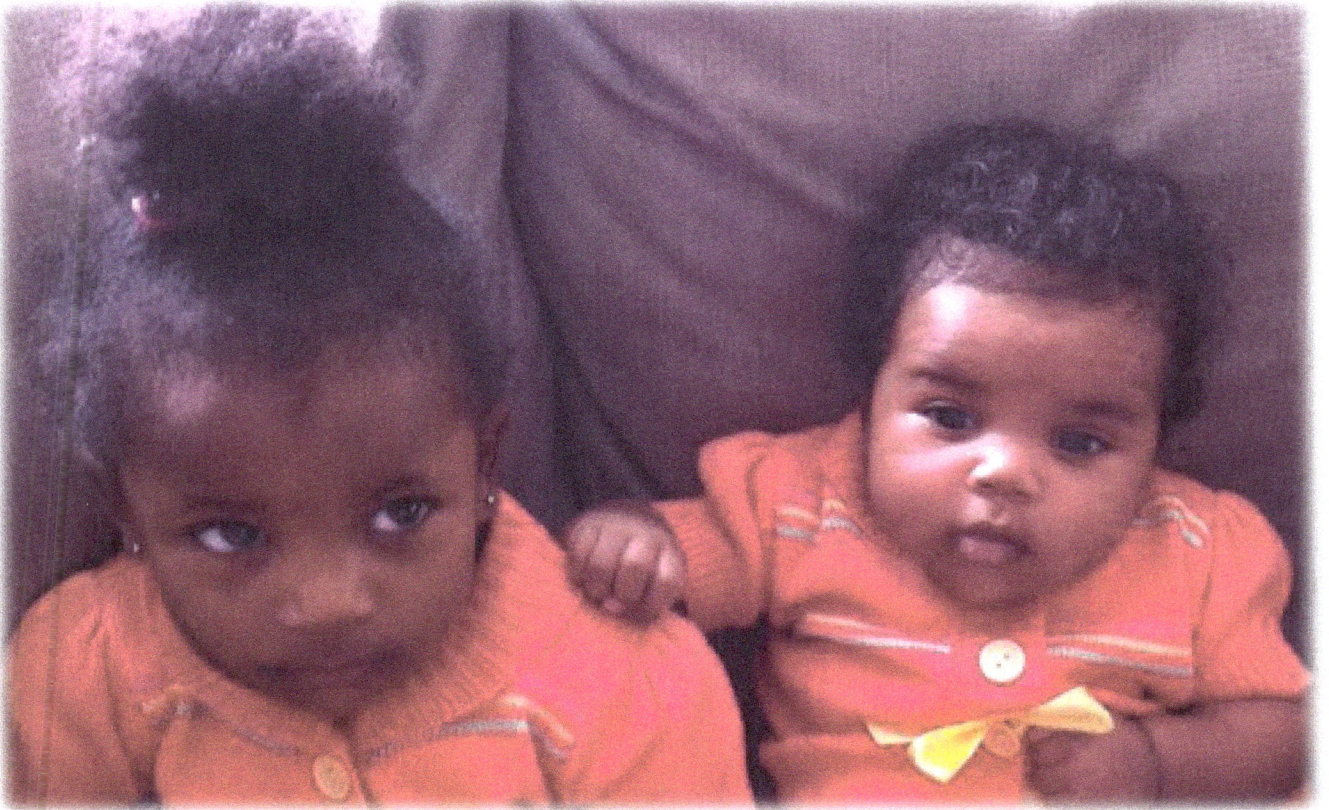

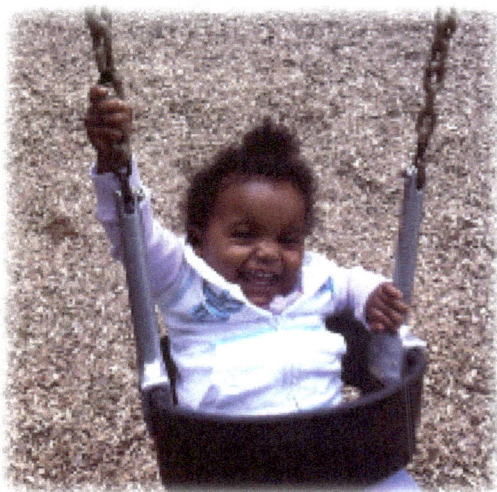

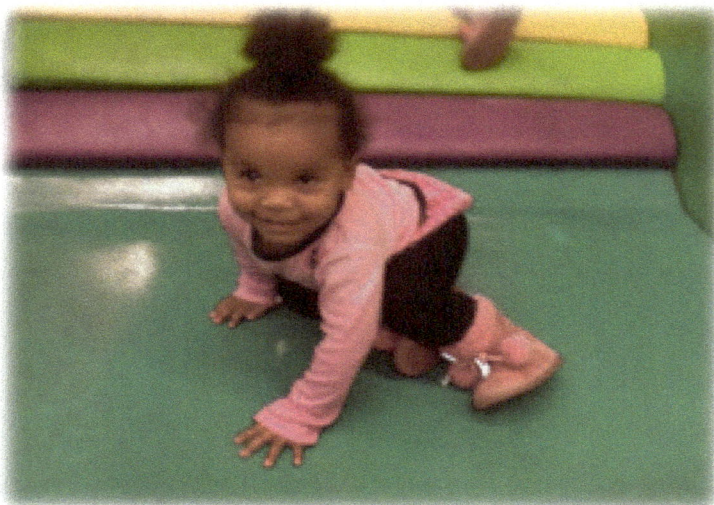

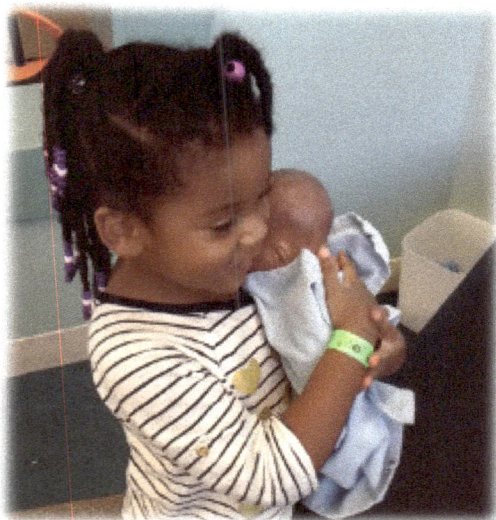

Juliana was walking, playing, and doing things, just like kids her age.

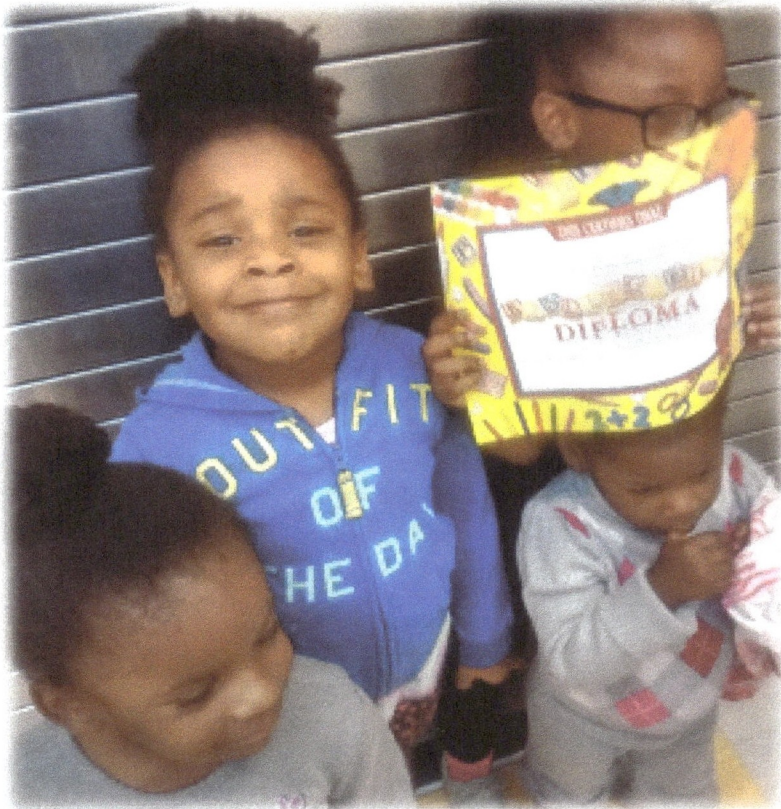

As Juliana got older, her father and I noticed that her speech was not very clear. At times, we understood her younger siblings Jael and Joella, more than we understood her.

That made us realize that this was not something she would grow out of without help.

Juliana would get frustrated when she had to repeat herself, so others could try to understand what she said. Many times she would say, "forget it." She didn't know why she had a challenge that none of her siblings did. We would encourage her to talk, even if we didn't always understand.

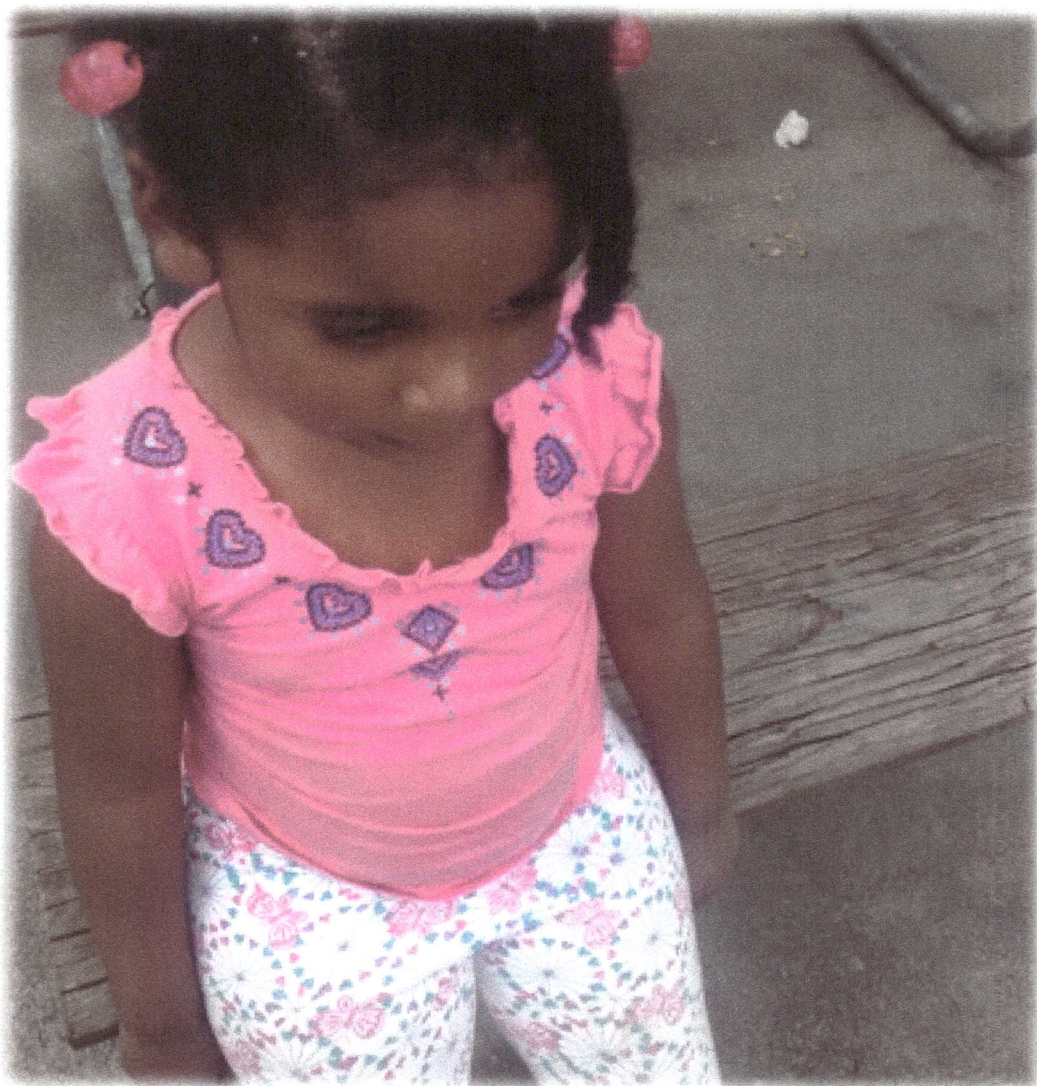

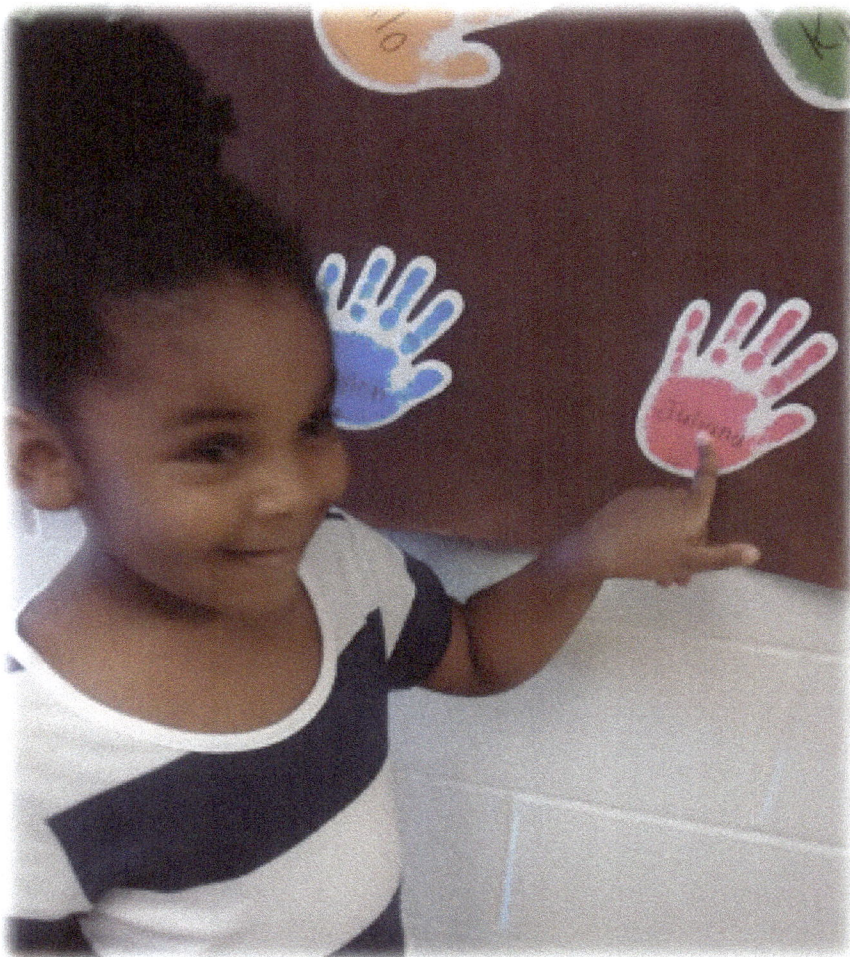

After speaking with her pediatrician about our concerns with Juliana's speech, she got a hearing test done, with no problems detected. Later, she had an assessment at school, confirming she would need speech therapy.

She began seeing a speech pathologist at her school in kindergarten. She started with a score of 58 on the Goldman-Fristoe Test of Articulation-3.

According to her first assessment, she initially had errors in speech sounds with K, G, J, CH, and consonant clusters. She participated in an Individualized Education Program (IEP) due to her speech. However, Juliana made great improvements that first year! She completed kindergarten in 2017.

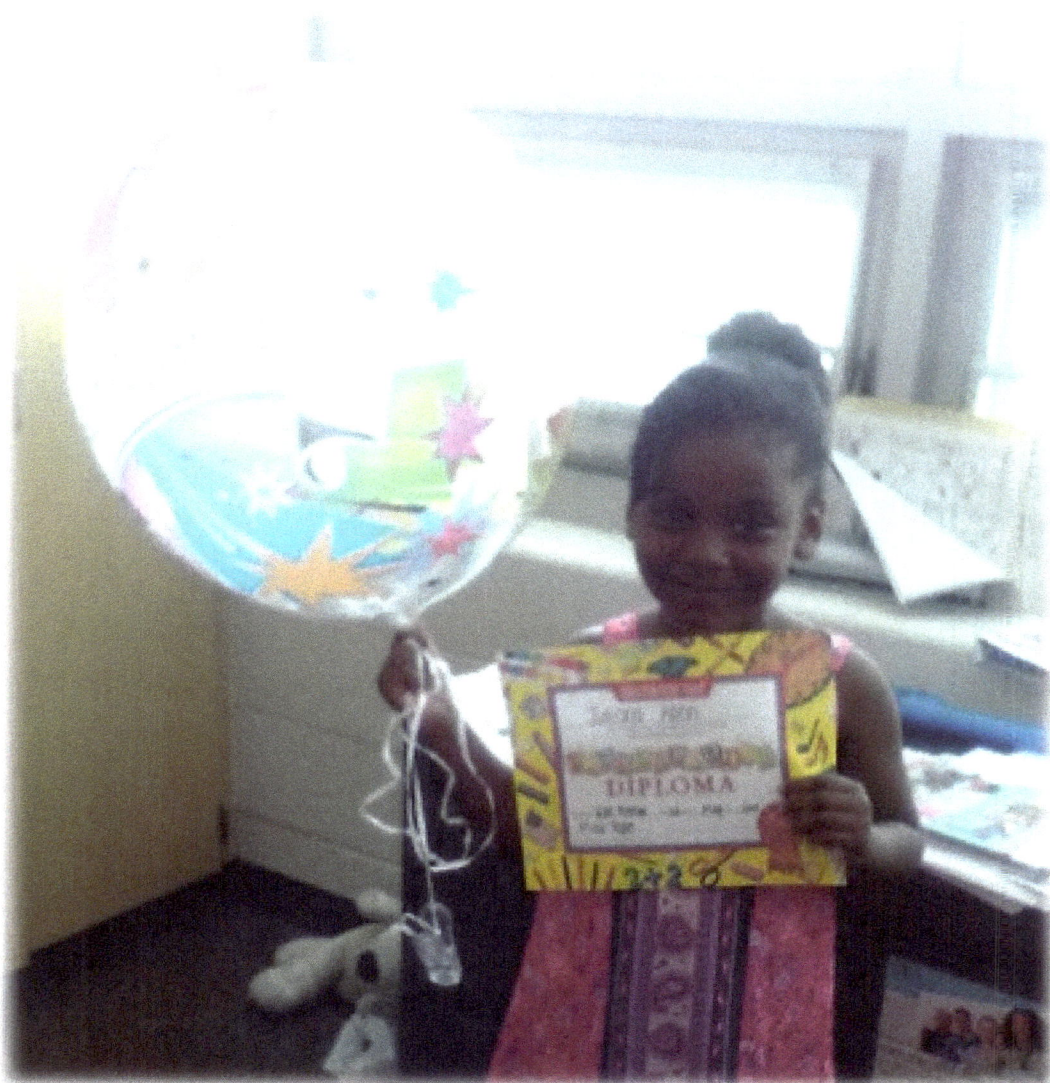

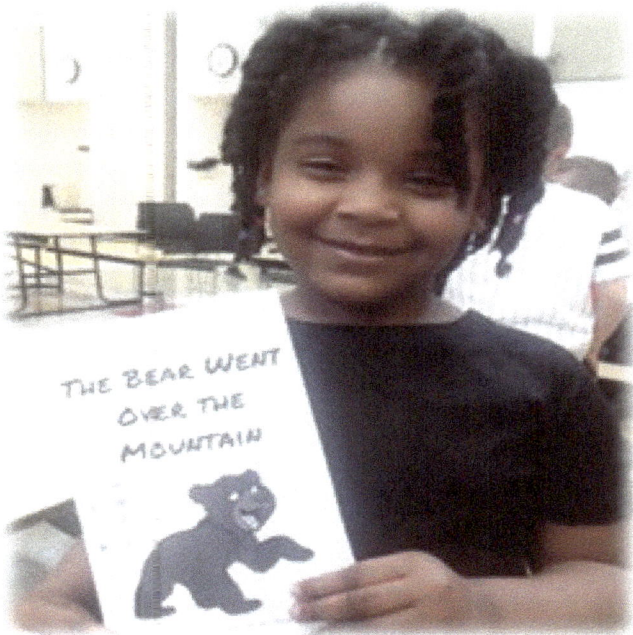

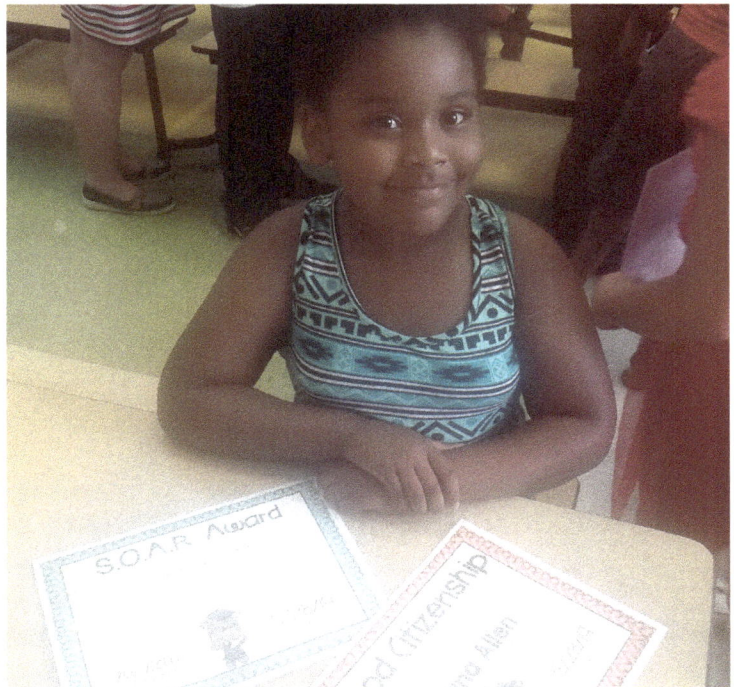

The success continued throughout her first- and second-grade years. Her confidence improved too! Go, Juliana!

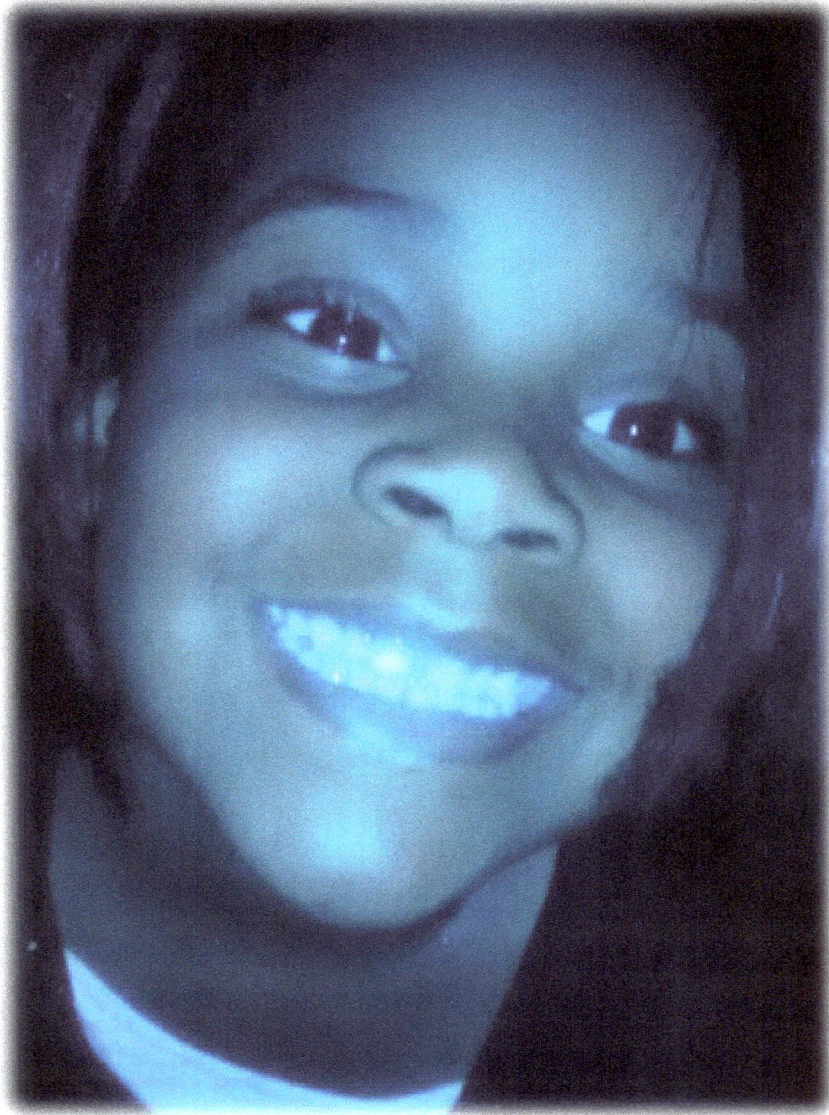

She began speaking more clearly as she worked hard at home and school on her speech. Juliana had activities, flashcards, books, and worksheets to help along the way.

Juliana was soon earning straight A's on spelling tests and volunteering to answer questions in class. She loves science and math!

Third grade came along with a pleasant surprise.
Juliana's assessment score jumped to 110!
She no longer needed speech therapy!

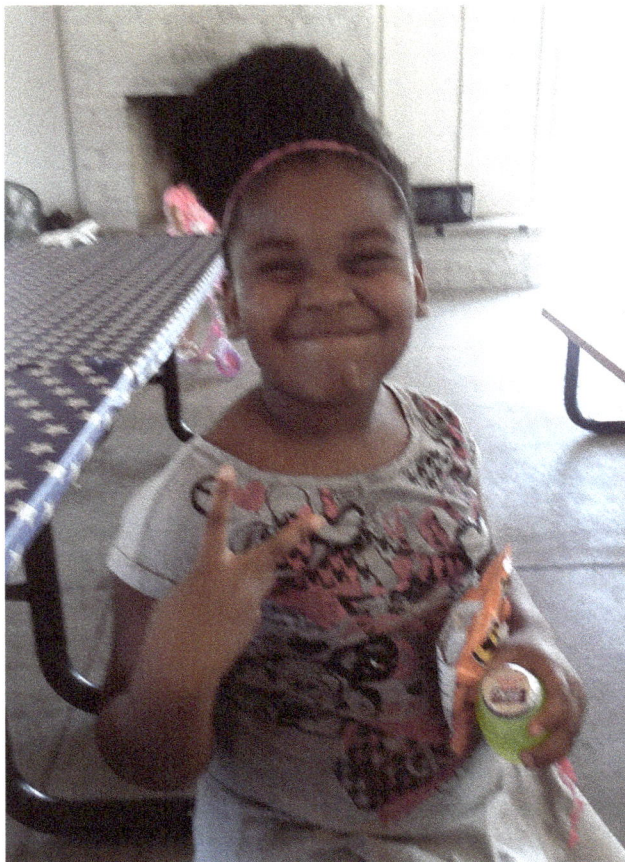

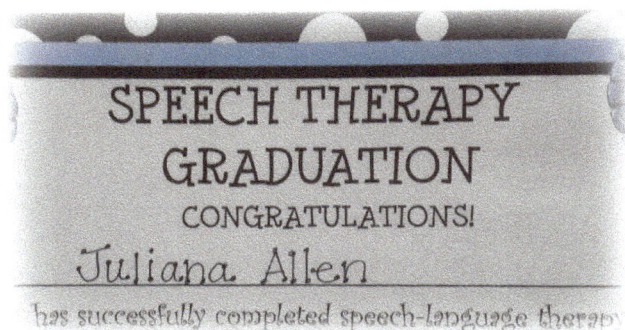

SPEECH THERAPY
GRADUATION
CONGRATULATIONS!
Juliana Allen
has successfully completed speech-language therapy

An Interview With Juliana

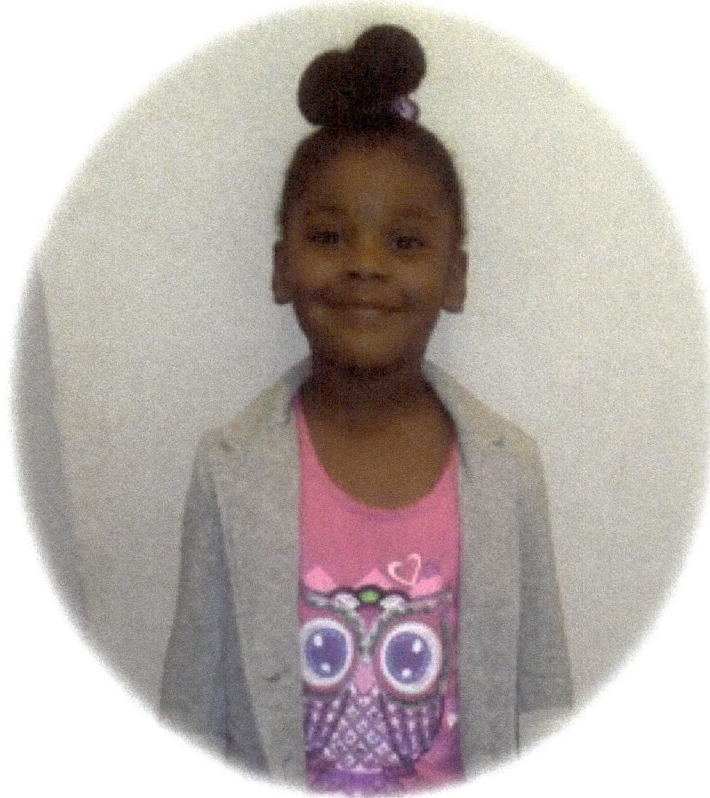

Q: What was getting speech therapy like?
A: "It was kind of fun, and we got to play with stuff. We would do words, and we would get timed on quizzes, and it was hard to say some words, but sometimes not."

Q: How did it make you feel?
A: "It made me feel better to be in a class like that. I got better and better, and I got to play more than doing timed quizzes. I got a sticker on a paper, and if I got all the way up to 20, I got a surprise."

Q: What would you tell other kids in speech therapy?
A: "I would tell them to try and try and try, and they will get better and better if they will just try."

Q: Should they feel bad about needing help?
A: "No, they shouldn't feel bad because if they do, they may not think they will get better, but they will."

Q: How old are you now?
A: "I am 8 years old."

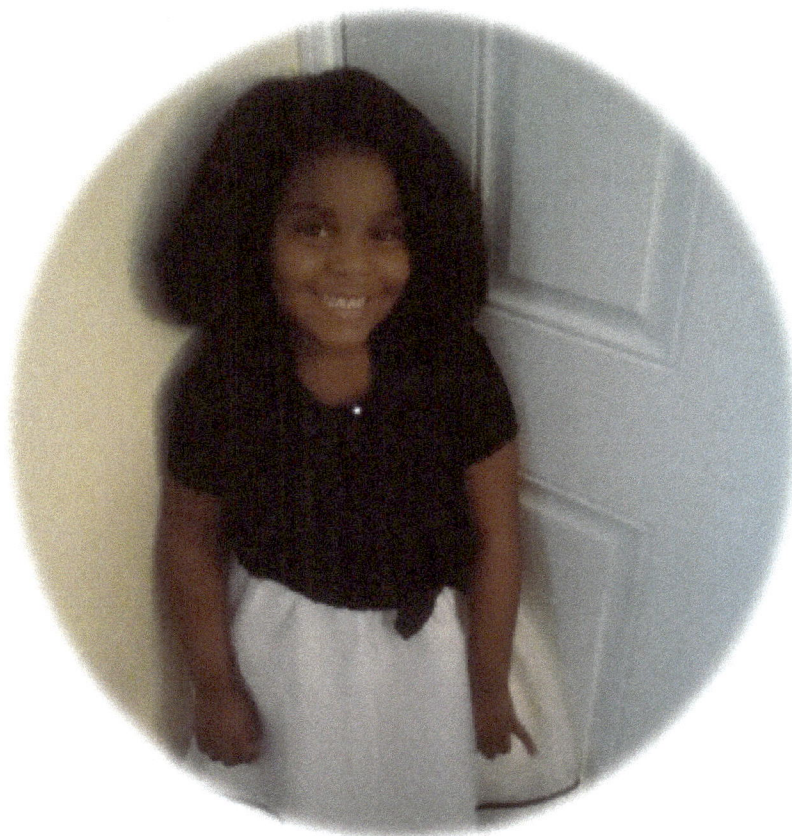

www.ingramcontent.com/pod-product-compliance
Lightning Source LLC
Chambersburg PA
CBHW051312020426
42333CB00027B/3308